ADHD and Teens

Natural Treatment for the ADHD Child

Haphiza Baboolal

Disclaimer

Care has been taken to ensure that the information in this eBook is accurate to the best of my knowledge. The reader should understand that the information provided in this eBook does not contain legal, medical or any kind of professional advice.

Just to let you know that I am neither a doctor nor do I consider myself to be one. I am not liable for mis- statements, omissions or inaccurate information. This book is for informational use only and does not guarantee that by using any of this information your child will be free from ADD/ADHD symptoms.

Should you choose to use any of this information for yourself, your child or anyone else I recommend you do so by first consulting with your medical practitioner? This product has no warranties. Following the suggestions in this book is done at your own risk.

The information provided in this eBook is not intended to substitute for medical advice from a health care professional. Please consult your doctor if you have any symptoms stated in this eBook or suffer from any medical condition. This eBook should not be used for diagnosing or treating health problems.

The author and publisher shall have neither responsibility nor liability to any person or entity with respect to any damage caused or alleged to be caused directly or indirectly by this eBook.

No liability: This product is supplied "as is" and without warranties. If you do not agree with the liability then please do not use or distribute this product.

No liability will be assumed for any losses or damages resulting directly or indirectly from the use of this product.

Contents

Introduction

The information in this eBook will help you the parents and or caregivers decide whether you want to give medications to your child who has many side effects such as: insomnia, loss of appetite, nausea, vomiting, weight gain, tics, allergic reaction, dizziness and many more. There are some drugs which do not work at all as was the case with my grandson.

Many parents do not want to give drugs to their children but do not know what else to do. If your child is already on medication please do not stop the medications before consulting your doctor, most of all if you stop the medications suddenly your child may encounter side effects or other problems.
Some children on the other hand do well with the medications and encounter very few side effects.

In the section **"Treatment Options for ADHD"** you will find several natural therapies diet changes, behavior interventions and other options that are worth looking into that can help your child.

You will learn what is ADHD, the signs and

symptoms of ADHD, its cause and how to get the most from the Education System to help your child.

My Encounter with ADHD

My grandchild who I will call Master K. has been living with me and my husband since birth. He was born a happy healthy lovable baby just like most babies. When he was just a few weeks old I noticed something strange was happening. He was having seizure like activities which the doctor was not concerned about and said it was normal movements even though I knew better.

Then later on I noticed he had problems with pronouncing his words properly and was stuttering. Again the doctor words were when he starts school and start mixing with other children his speech will get better.

He entered pre-k and things got even worse till he had to be seen by a psychiatrist .After evaluating him, a diagnosis of ADHD made with possibly Tourettes Syndrome and Pervasive Developmental Disorder (PDD).

Since I had never heard of such a health problem I listened to the doctors and put him on medications. Some medications would work for a few weeks and some did not. So the struggles dealing with this child continued.

As time went by I started researching and learning more about ADHD and Tourettes Syndrome. He is now 14 years old and at this time his tics from the Tourettes Syndrome almost do not exist except when he gets angry.

I started him on Omega-3 fish oils which he is still taking, I tried several other vitamins and minerals and a few other things sold at the health food store that they said would help. Nothing had worked. He has had counseling at school for several years from Pre-K to 8th grade and it had not helped.

He is now finishing Middle School and is still facing behavior issues which he is being seen by a Counselor from outside the school. He has only had 5 sessions from this counselor and even though the change is very small he has progressed more than all the years of counseling he has had in schools.

So if you find that the counseling your child is getting at school is not helping, don't be afraid to find a counselor from outside the school. Ask friends or your church members or just people you meet and if they know of someone they will surely tell you.

If you don't have health insurance you can apply

2

for Medicaid help for your child. I know having health insurance is a big problem for a lot of people but there is a lot of help out there. When you don't get the help you need from one person keep going until you get the help that your child needs.

I know how frustrated you are with getting help for your child because I have been there. No one knows your child better than you do. Therefore I urge you if you think there is something wrong with your child and your doctor wants to shrug it off, change your doctor and keep looking until you find someone to help you and your child. Find someone who will listen to you and work with you.

You just have to find the right doctor to work with you whether you medicate your child or use alternative medicine.

What is ADHD?

ADHD stands for Attention Deficit Hyperactivity Disorder.
There is also ADD.

ADD stands for Attention Deficit Disorder. The child or adult does not have the hyperactivity.

ADHD is one of the most common neurobehavioral disorders of childhood which affects different parts of the brain. 3-5% of American children are affected by this disorder. ADHD is often times mis-diagnosed and treatment not always effective although some children have had good results.

The condition is frustrating for the child, the parent and the rest of the family. Teachers, physicians and other healthcare professionals become frustrated, as well. To achieve the best results, everyone in the child's environment needs to work together. My goal here is to help you understand the condition and treatment options.

The most common symptoms of ADHD are impulsiveness, hyperactivity and inattention. Your child may not have all of these behavioral problems. Some kids are just hyperactive. Others get sidetracked, daydream or become bored, when they should be learning new skills.

It interferes with a person's ability to stay on task.
It is usually first diagnosed in childhood and often lasts
into adulthood.

ADD/ADHD does not discriminate. It can affect
anyone rich or poor of any race regardless if you
live in the best part of town or not.

Understanding ADHD

We all have difficulty sitting still, controlling impulse behavior or paying attention at times. But for children and adults the problem is such that it interferes with their lives at home, school, work and socially.

Children with ADD, ADHD can be very successful in life if the problem is identified and treated. If the problem is not identified it can have serious consequences in the life of that individual.

They may have behavioral problems, failing in school, unable to make and keep friends, considered to be a trouble maker, find themselves in gangs and doing drugs, have failed relationships.

So identifying and treating these problems are very important for the child and the family members. If these individuals are not diagnosed and treated the disorder will continue into adulthood and there will be consequences at work and in their marriage lives.

6

It was believed that children outgrew ADHD in adolescence because their hyperactivity became less. However most of the symptoms continue into adulthood. When the adult does not know how to deal with the situation they become very anxious and depressed.

Children with ADD/ADHD may feel that they are different from other children their own age and sometimes they are made fun of at school. When this happens the teacher or someone who knows more about ADD/ADHD should explain to the children in simple terms what ADD/ADHD is all about. Some children are very knowledgeable about ADD/ADHD and can explain to the class what it is.

When other children understand what a person is going through they become less mean and often help that person instead. ADHD is over diagnosed and over treated.

The child who has been diagnosed with ADD/ADHD has brain that goes like a speeding car without the brakes working properly. They have trouble putting the brakes on everything.

Data & Statistics from the Centers for Disease Control and Prevention

In the United States

- 4.5 million Children 5-17 years of age have ever been diagnosed with ADHD as of 2006.

- 7.8% of school-aged children were reported to have an ADHD diagnosis by their parent in 2003.

- Diagnosis of ADHD increased an average of 3% per year from 1997 to 2006.

- Boys (9.5%) are more likely than girls (5.9%) to have been diagnosed with ADHD.

- Diagnosed cases of attention deficit hyperactivity disorder increased almost 4 percent every year from 2000 to 2010 making it the number one mental health concern in children.

- Boys are twice as likely to be diagnosed as girls. This is down dramatically from the 10 to 1 ratio in 1997.

- It is estimated that 3-5% of school-aged children

are affected by ADHD.

- Diagnosed cases of attention deficit hyperactivity disorder increased almost 4 percent every year from 2000 to 2010 making it the number one mental health concern in children.

- Currently 60 percent of all children with ADHD are receiving medication for treating the disorder, with Ritalin continuing to be the most widely prescribed.

- The most highly medicated age demographic for ADHD children are those from 9 to 12 years of age.

- In America, the state with highest number of cases reported was Alabama with the highest number of prescriptions being written in Arkansas.

Research suggests that this condition is an imbalance or deficiency in brain chemicals that regulates inattention/distractibility, impulsive behavior, and hyperactivity or restlessness which begins before the age of 7, but most of the time will continue into the teenage years and adulthood.

Signs and Symptoms of ADHD in Children

Children with ADHD have trouble with:

Inattention, hyperactivity, and impulsivity which are the key behaviors of ADHD. It is normal for all children to be inattentive, hyperactive, or impulsive sometimes, but for children with ADHD, these behaviors are more severe and occur more often. To be diagnosed with the disorder, a child must have symptoms for 6 or more months, starts before age 7 and to a degree that is greater than other children of the same age.

Symptoms of inattention

•   Paying attention, these children are easily distracted, forget things, forget details and often switch from one activity to another without completing any.

•   Controlling impulsive behaviors (may act without thinking about what the result will be), and in some cases, are overly active.

•   Have difficulty focusing

Difficulty with organizing

- Unless they are doing something they enjoy they become bored very easily. They do not seem to listen when spoken to.

- Daydream and become confused easily.

- Very forgetful, struggle to follow instructions.

- Trouble completing homework and turning it in.

- Always losing things (e.g., pencils, books, toys assignments.)

Children who have symptoms of hyperactivity may:

- Fidget and squirm in their seats

- Talk nonstop

- Dash around, touching or playing with anything and everything in sight

- Have trouble sitting still during dinner, school, and story time

- Be constantly in motion

- Have difficulty doing quiet tasks or activities.

Children who have symptoms of impulsivity may:

- Be very impatient.

- Blurt out inappropriate comments, show their emotions without restraint, and act without regard for consequences

- Have difficulty waiting for things they want or waiting their turns in games.

- Often interrupt conversations or others' activities.

These children are often picky eaters only eating 2 or 3 types of food, and have trouble sleeping.

What Causes ADHD?

Genes may play a large role in someone being diagnosed with ADHD although there are several other factors that may play a large part. As with many other disabilities, there is no one explanation that can be given for why a child or adult has a learning disability. Many factors may be responsible for learning disabilities.

Some researchers believe that learning disabilities result from complications that occur before, during, or shortly after birth. Males are more likely to have a learning disability than females. Learning disabilities tend to occur in families. So if a parent has ADHD it is likely that one or more of their children will have ADHD.

According to the National Institute of Mental Health

Scientists are not sure what causes ADHD, although many studies suggest that genes play a large role. Like so many other illnesses, ADHD probably results from a number of factors including genetics. Researchers are also looking at environmental factors, and are studying how brain injuries, nutrition, and the social environment might contribute to ADHD.

Genes. Genes are the blueprint we inherit from our

parents. Studies show that ADHD often runs in families. Researchers are looking at several genes that may make people more likely to develop the disorder.

Environmental factors. Studies suggest there may be a link between cigarette smoking and alcohol use during pregnancy and ADHD in children. Scientists are studying the use of alcohol during pregnancy. Children also inhale whatever is in the environment or in the air and it get into the lungs of these children.

Chemicals

Chemicals are also found in the carpets in your homes, upholstery, rugs, mattresses, soaps and toothpaste and the list goes on. Chemicals are also found on the clothes that you dry clean.

Additives, Coloring and Dyes

Many people believe that additives, coloring and dyes contribute to hyperactivity and inattention.

There have been a lot of studies on the effects of artificial food dyes on children, dating back to the 1970s. Some showed that food dyes could cause behavioral problems in children, and others didn't.

Studies suggest that when certain dyes and coloring are removed from the diet the symptoms were reduced.

Preservatives

Some parents and caregivers believe that preservatives have a negative effect on some children's behavior which can affect their ability to learn. You may want to cut out preservatives from your child diet for a period of time and monitor if there was a negative effect or not.

The issue is controversial with experts offering at times opposing views at times.

Food Sensitivities

A large number of children who have been diagnosed with ADHD may be sensitive to eating certain foods, which may be the primary cause of their ADHD. This response may be the primary cause of their ADHD. In what type of child should you suspect food allergies?

Here is a list of some symptoms that may result from food sensitivities in certain children:

Hyperactivity

- Changes in mood

- Halitosis

- Sleep disturbances

- Delay in sleep onset

- Migraines

- Other headaches

- Abdominal pain

- Bedwetting

- Tantrums

- Eczema

- Asthma

- Seizures

Research shows that by treating the food allergies all of these symptoms can be relieved.

If you see your child's symptoms in this list it is possible that food allergies may be contributing to his problem. If your child has allergies such as asthma then food allergies most certainly will be contributing to their problem.

You may want to have your child tested for food allergies or you can play detective and try to figure out what your child is allergic to by eliminating a certain food for a period of about two weeks and observe them.

Gluten Free Diet

In a small study, children with ADHD had been put on a Gluten free diet, foods that are free of gluten such as acorn, amaranth, garbanzo, beans, brown rice and buckwheat. Behavior changes had improved and the children had an increased attention span and were able to focus better.

Sulfites are sulfur-based compounds that may be added to foods as an enhancer and preservative. Sulfites can also be found in cooked and processed foods. Always read food labels to check for sulfites.

Some sulfite-containing ingredients to look for on food labels include:

- Sulfur dioxide

- Potassium bisulfite or potassium metabisulfite
- Sodium bisulfite, sodium metabisulfite, or sodium sulfite

Some foods that contain sulfites include:

- Baked goods
- Pickled foods
- Dried fruits
- Canned vegetables
- Trail mix
- Teas
- Soup mixes

Be sure to read labels.

Mono Sodium Glutamate (MSG)

Monosodium glutamate enhances the flavor of food and is add to foods like canned vegetables, so I would avoid canned foods, processed meats such as hot dogs and cold cuts, Chinese food, soy sauce and other foods.

MSG is also contained in additives that say:

- Calciun caseinate

- Sodiun caseinate

- Autolyzed yeast

- Anything hydrolyzed

When eating at restaurants ask if their foods contain MSG if it does contain MSG ask if they can leave it out of your food.

Pesticides

Pesticides are a common concern especially outside the home and on the food that our children eat. Pesticides are toxic and our children eat it, our food is sprayed with it, and it is also used to kill bugs and insects and spray the lawns. Children eat these foods and play on the lawn which they then absorb these toxins.

Preschoolers are exposed to high levels of lead which are found in old plumbing fixtures or paint in old buildings. These children have a higher risk of developing ADHD because small children tend to bite on the edges of and swallow the paint.

Sugar. A lot of people got the idea that using refined sugar makes the ADHD child hyper-activity worse.

Research does not support this.

Food additives. Recent British research indicates a possible link between consumption of certain food additives like artificial colors or preservatives. Research is under way to confirm the findings and to learn more about how food additives may affect hyperactivity.

Scientist is also studying the use of alcohol and tobacco during pregnancy.

Characteristics

Sometimes parents and other caregivers who work with young ones with learning disabilities may think the child is just lazy, spoiled, daydreaming, bored or is not disciplined.

Some of the most common characteristics are as follows:

- Short attention span/easily distracted

- Poor memory/forgetful

- Difficulty following directions

- Poor reasoning ability

- Inability to set realistic goals

- Poor reading ability (e.g., adds, omits, skips words when reading)

- Difficulty distinguishing between p, g, b, d, and q

- Reads "on" for "no", "was" for "saw", etc.

- Difficulty with concepts left-right, above-below, up-down, yesterday-tomorrow, in-out, etc.

- Difficulty telling time

- Difficulty writing

- Poor eye-hand coordination

- Clumsy/accident prone

- Disorganized/loses things

- Quick tempered/easily irritated

- Impulsive

- Gets caught up in details

- Childish and bossy behavior

- Needs constant recognition

- A loner

Some of these children are also very bright and can read very well. When it comes to writing this is a big problem for most of them, their writing is very sloppy and they themselves cannot understand it.

Lucky for computers some children can even do their work using computers instead of writing which makes it easier on the child and also for the caregivers.

Can Other Problems Be Mistaken For ADHD

Many children have mistakenly been diagnosed as having ADHD because there are several health problems that mimic some of the same signs and symptoms.

There is no test for making a diagnosis of ADHD. Tests are based on using standard guidelines from the American Academy of Pediatrics. A diagnosis is made by gathering information from the child parents or caregiver.

A child has to show some or all the symptoms on a regular basis for at least 6 months in 2 or more settings such as at school and at home. Both the parents and teacher or caregivers are asked to complete the questioners about the child's behavior and environment.

Many pediatricians will refer the child to see a mental health specialist who is experienced in childhood disorders. The doctors will try to rule out any other possibilities that may have these symptoms.

Physical and medical history.

A physical is taken to screen for visual or hearing problems, allergies, seizures and eczema which can all produce symptoms that mimic ADHD. You may have to ask your doctor to perform these tests some of them will but some of them would not.

There are also other conditions that can affect a child's behavior such as:
- Mood disorders
- Thyroid disorders
- Anxiety disorders
- Lead toxicity
- Sleep dysfunction
- Parasites
- Chemical imbalance

When a child is diagnosed with ADHD there are normally other health problems that exist including:
- Tourettes Syndrome
- Learning disorders
- Behavioral issues
- Oppositional defiant disorder (ODD)
- Anxiety
- Depression

So a child with ADHD may have more to deal with other than just the ADHD.

Learning Disability

Alfred A. Strauss, M.D. is the first person to describe the behaviors of children and adults now identified as learning disability. These adults and children are not mentally retarded but some of them are very intelligent.

An individual with learning disability, the message to the brain becomes jumbled which makes it difficult for the individual to learn in one or more academic area. Despite this problem some of these individuals become very successful.

Some of these individuals who had learning disabilities were Thomas Edison, Albert Einstein, Nelson Rockefeller, Winston Churchill and many others. Many of them found a different approach to learning from how most people learn. Research shows that individuals with learning disabilities that go undetected do not do well in school.

The National Center for Learning Disabilities (http://www.ncld.org/) lists some words commonly associated with learning disabilities that will be helpful as you work with youth with learning disabilities.

- Dyslexia, perhaps the most commonly known, is

primarily used to describe difficulty with language processing and its impact on reading, writing, and spelling.

- Dysgraphia involves difficulty with writing. Problems might be seen in the actual motor patterns used in writing. Also characteristic are difficulties with spelling and the formulation of written composition.

- Dyscalculia involves difficulty with math skills and impacts math computation. Memory of math facts, concepts of time, money, and musical concepts can also be impacted.

- Dyspraxia (Apraxia) is a difficulty with motor planning, and impacts upon a person's ability to coordinate appropriate body movements.

- Auditory Discrimination is a key component of efficient language use, and is necessary to "break the code" for reading. It involves being able to perceive the differences between speech sounds, and to sequence these sounds into meaningful words.

- Visual Perception is critical to the reading and writing processes as it addresses the ability to

27

notice important details and assign meaning to what is seen.

- Attention Deficit (Hyperactivity) Disorder (ADD/ADHD) may co-occur with learning disabilities (incidence estimates vary). Features can include: marked over-activity, distractibility, and/or impulsivity which in turn can interfere with an individual's availability to benefit from instruction.

My Child Has Been Diagnosed with ADHD. What's next?

Parents who have just been given the diagnosis that their child has ADHD get very confused and has a lot of questions, concerns and they sometimes deny the diagnosis.

Your child has been diagnosed with ADHD. It may be a relief in some ways, to put a name with the issues you have been dealing with. One decision parents have to contemplate, which is rather large a decision, is whether to medicate or not medicate their child who is struggling with ADHD. There is no right or wrong answer. The decision to medicate or not needs to be addressed on an individual basis by the family and caretakers.

You need to talk this over with your significant other, family members, caretakers etc. You may also want to talk to other parents that you know who may have children or know someone that may have children with ADHD to get their input. The bottom line is only you can make that decision.

There are times when you may need to start your child off with medication while looking for alternative treatments if that is your goal. If your child had diabetes would you not him/her medications to control their diabetes.

There are several treatment options to choose from therefore parents, doctors, therapists, counselors and other caregivers should work together for the benefit of the child. You are your child's advocate so make use of all the resources available to you and your child.

Parents should attend a parental training course which will help them to deal with issues that will arise from their child's behavior.

A good treatment plan will include close monitoring of the child with follow ups and any changes that may be needed.

Treatment options for ADHD

- Medications
- Alternative therapy
- Behavioral interventions

- Education

- Nature

- Swimming

- Education

- Nature

- Swimming

- Transformation Program

The decision to medicate or not medicate your child is a difficult one that you really have to think about.

If you choose to medicate your child have the doctor who is prescribing medications to let you know how the medication will affect your child. Any symptoms of drowsiness, poor appetite, difficulty in sleeping or eating if there are feeling nauseated and any other side effects that you should look for. How long the child should be on the medication before seeing any improvement. How long they may need to be on the medication.

Children tolerate medications differently so what may work for one child may not work for another. Sometimes the side effects of these medications such as Ritalin, Dexedrine and others may be worse than the child actual ADHD.

Getting the most from the education system:

Can My Child Be Given Medications at School?

Yes! Your child is allowed to take medications at school but a special form called a 504 form has to be completed by the doctor and then taken to the school nurse with the medications. The nurse will have the child come down to the nurse's office at the appropriate time to take their medication.

- This plan needs to be included in the child Individualized Education Program (IEP.)

- Need to maintain the child and parents right to confidentiality.

- Medications are to be administered in accordance with the rules of the facility.

We will discuss alternative therapies in more detail later on.

Behavioral therapy

Behavior therapy does help many children, but there must be clarity consistency and persistence for it to work. Do not expect results overnight, this may be a long process but all care givers have to chip in and help.

Make sure the child understands what you say to

him/her, you can also have your child repeat what you just said to make sure they understand the instructions that were given.

There should be consequences for appropriate and inappropriate behaviors. The child should understand which behaviors are acceptable and which are not. The behaviors you want to change in your child should be written down and put where the child can see it.

Do not try to change all the behaviors at the same time. Just work on one or two of the most important ones. If you try to make too many changes at the same time the child may become confused and frustrated and it will not work.

Education

Most children start school in regular classes. Many parents do not know that there is a problem with their child until they start school. If the teacher finds there is a problem they will call the parents to let them know their child has not been paying attention, constantly moving around when they should be sitting, blurting out answers, difficulty focusing, daydreaming etc.

With the classes in most schools with over 30 children to teach most teachers put pressure on parents to have their child seen by their doctor to either put them on medications to calm them in the class room or to rule out ADHD. With such large classes the teachers find it impossible to deal with these children and teach at the same time because some of these children are very disruptive.

Most children do not do well in the education system because they need extra attention and disrupt the class. A lot of parents home school their children because the child cannot keep up with the work at school.

If you think your child has a problem with hyperactivity or attention or having a problem with learning you can request the school to perform an assessment for your child. Schools are required to perform this assessment if you request it. This is a free service performed by the school.

You can choose whether your child goes to a public school, private school or whether you home school your child. If you have placed your child in a private school, or if your child's school does not receive federal funding, you may not have access to many of the services and accommodations offered in public schools.

Parents can relate to those who are doing the assessment the type of educational difficulties their child is having.

The school cannot make a diagnosis only a trained health professional can diagnose a child.

The child has to be accurately diagnosed by a knowledgeable well trained clinician. Most parents fear the word ADHD and go into denial. With the proper diagnosis there is a lot of help you can find for your child.

The doctor may want to try your child on medications; several different medications may need to be tried before finding one that will actually help your child. So you need to be very patient.

Should your child need to take medications during school hours a special form is filled out (a form called 504) and has to be signed by the doctor so the child can be given their medications during school hours.

The child may also be assigned to a special education class in which they are taught their lessons in a much smaller classroom setting. This way the child can get individual attention and work at a pace that is comfortable for him/her.

For children who are younger than 5 years old you may want to contact Early Childhood Programs that are specialized with helping the little ones with disabilities.

These children learn best in a structure environment whether at home or at school. The rules and expectations should be clear and consistent ahead of time and consequences delivered immediately.

The rules and regulations should be explained in simple terms that the child can understand using short sentences and having the child repeat what was just said so they understand.

Accommodations for helping the child

The following may be helpful:

- Speak short sentences so the child understands and have them repeat what you just said.
- Setting specific times for specific tasks, these children do not deal with changes too well. They need a routine.
- When you have to change anything from their routine let them know ahead of time.
- Make a daily schedule with any assignments.
- Have a quiet space for the child to work.

- Have them sit at the front of the class where there is less distraction away from doors and windows.
- Provide frequent breaks.
- They may want to stand or sit on the floor to do their class work because they feel more comfortable that way.
- Using visual instructions instead of verbal instructions.
- Using computer for learning.
- Need to be taught organizational skills.
- Modifying test time.

The ADHD Child At Home

Caring for a child with ADD/ADHD is very challenging for both parents and siblings. Parents often do not know how to deal with these children. When they have a behavior problem the parents become overwhelmed because other siblings get punched at and tortured. There are some children who argue a lot, are defiant, refuse to pay attention or follow instructions which can cause havoc in the home.

Sometimes parents pamper these children and instead of disciplining the child they make all sorts of excuses which do not help the child. Some parents do not know what to do or where to go for help. They watch as their family fall apart and the child controls the household.

Often parents feel that they are to be blamed for their child ADHD or think that they are not good parents and so feel ashamed to seek help. Some parents blame each other for allowing the child to get away with poor behavior and the other may think it is too harsh.

You as a parent can take control and help your child and your family. It will be hard work but it can be done. You will need to set up a support system to help you.

From time to time most children can be difficult to deal with but a child with ADHD is even more challenging which can make parents feel alone and isolated.

- Meet other parents that are going through the same situation. Ask the social worker if they can help you find a support group if you don't know of any.

- Visit www.chadd.org they can help you locate a CHADD Chapter near where you live.

- If possible have a friend or relative who will be willing to look after your child even for a few hours so you can get a break and not be overwhelmed.

Parental training will help you to:

- Set up methods that teach and reward children for appropriate behavior and give time out or loss privileges for inappropriate behavior.

- Provide clear expectations and directions so the child will understand. Caregivers do not always specify what is expected of the child and when the child does not meet that expectation they think the child has failed.

- Focus on one or two goals at a time. Focusing on too many goals will overwhelm the child and get them frustrated.

- Help your child learn from his/her mistakes. Explain in simple terms what your child did right or wrong. Praise you child when they do something right or something nice.

- Let your child know that you love them even though you may not believe this sometimes. Your child is going through a difficult time and so are you. Let your child know that you will get through this together.

- Even though your child may not have social skills you can learn how to help your child make friends and how to handle it.

- Your ADHD child may be having some issues with education but he/she may be very athletic, be skillful in computers, art, painting or even music. Help the child develop those skills so they will have a great sense of pride and accomplishment. Do not withhold these skills as a form of punishment for misbehaving.

- Spend some special time with your child alone whether it is to read a book or play a game of tic tac toe or just a walk outside.

Sleep and the ADHD Child

There are many reasons why children have problems falling asleep occasionally but children with ADD/ADHD have a lot of difficult falling asleep. Some medications may cause your child not to be able to fall asleep. Others just cannot fall asleep either because they are too busy thinking about other things or just cannot get to sleep.

When my grandchild was much smaller he would say to us that he wished night did not exist so that he would not have to go to sleep. Remember he also was diagnosed with ADHD and Tourettes Syndrome.

Helping Your ADHD Child to Sleep

There are some things we can do to help our children sleep.

- If medications are keeping your child awake at night talk the child's doctor to see if the medication can be changed.

- Try to keep your child schedule with limited changes if possible. I know the kids says it is vacation time and I should be able to stay up later when this happens and school reopens you would be faced with a lot of problems.

- Keep their bedtime routine the same and have them wake up the same time each day. Children need consistency.

- Some children find their creative juices start flowing as soon they put their heads on their pillow and this keeps them awake.

- Music works well with some children. Music such as Jazz or Mozart is very good.

- There are CD's with sounds such as rain, chirping of the birds, waterfall, waves or an electric fan are some things that can be used.

- Other things include a warm bath before going to bed, a foot massage, some lavender oil rubbed on the temples, burning some essential oils or spraying some orange essential oils on their pillows.

- Avoid caffeine in beverages and snacks after about 5pm.

- Avoid games such as video games, play station and other stimulating games before bedtime also avoid physical activities a few hours before bedtime.

- For younger children you can read them a bedtime story or just tell a story that the child will enjoy tuck them in and give then a good night kiss and let them know that you love them.

- Sometimes listening to relaxing music help calm the child and they fall asleep.

Can Children With ADHD Get Better?

Children with ADHD can get better with treatment, but there is no cure. There are three basic types of treatment:

- **Medication**. Several medications can help. The most common types are called stimulants. Medications help children focus, learn, and stay calm. Some parents do not want to use medications because they do not like the side effects others think the older children will get hooked on it.

- Sometimes medications cause side effects, such as sleep problems or stomachaches. Your child may need to try a few medications to see which one works best. It's important that you and your doctor watch your child closely while he or she is taking medicine.

- **Therapy**. There are different kinds of therapy. Behavioral therapy can help teach children to control their behavior so they can do better at school and at home.

- **Medication and therapy combined**.
  Some parents may prefer to combine medication and therapy at the same time.

ADHD and Teenagers

Most teens with ADHD are embarrassed with the diagnosis of having ADHD.

Many of them deny that they have ADHD because they may feel different from their friends. Teens are also facing other challenges at this time discovering their identity, dealing with peer pressure and other things that are going on in their lives.

They also need to focus on organization skills and academic issues. The teen should be told that having ADHD is not their fault nor is it caused by something they may have done.

Teens may also have poor self-esteem, feel stressed, tired and feel their parents did not understand them. They may also tell you there is nothing wrong with me. I am fine they may even refuse to take their medications.

Teen age years are very challenging for most parents, but the teenager with ADHD this is an even more trying time for them. They are now faced with trying to find their identity, schooling, trying to fit in with others, making and keeping new friends so for these children this is much harder for them to handle.

These children now desire to be independent and try doing things like using drugs, becoming sexually active and using alcohol which can lead to bad consequences. Don't forget at this time lots of teenagers are getting their drivers license and using their family vehicles. They pick up friends drink alcohol and speed the streets causing accidents.

Even though the teenager may be more capable in some ways, in other ways they need to have different rules and adhere to them. Both parents may not agree on what privileges the child may have and start fighting with each other so problems start occurring in the home.

The child should be given rules to adhere to and have consequences if the rules are broken. The rules should also be explained and the reason for the rule. Communication between parent and child is even more important now.

Rules should be posted on the refrigerator or in a convenient location so that the child knows it is there. These teenagers should be able to help with appropriate household chores and other things around the house also.

At this time the teenager will want to spend more time away from home with friends and just doing other things. They will want to demand later curfew and even the use of your vehicle. Listen to what your child is saying, you may also need to negotiate some of the request to come to a better understanding of helping your child to understand what you are relating.

They will resent certain restrictions but you have to be firm if you think it is in your child's best interest. Let them know the rules are to be carried out no matter what or there will be consequences.

These children sometimes become difficult and may not want to take their medications that are prescribed for them or they may not want to eat healthy cooked foods at home. They will want to consume a lot of fast foods to fill their stomachs which is not healthy for them.

Guide your child and try to understand what they are going through. Help them to make good choices. Avoid punishing your child every time he/she does something wrong or break the rules. Let your child know you are always there for them and they can come to you even if it is just to talk.

Even though the symptoms of ADHD may change as the child grows, teens with ADD/ADHD still require treatment and may need treatment into adulthood.

Depression and the ADHD Child

Depression is defined as an illness when the feelings of sadness, hopelessness, and despair persist and interfere with a child or adolescent's ability to function normally.

Some depression is normal in people lasts for a short period of time such as when a family member dies, or there is a divorce in the family. You freeze and don't know what to think or what to feel so you become numb and depressed. But this phase eventually passes as time goes by.

About 5% of adolescence and teenagers suffer from depression but the risk of a child with ADHD, learning and conduct disorders are much greater. Depression and ADHD can be treated with medications and behavior therapies.

Over time depression has become more common and is now recognized in younger children. Suicide rate in the teens increases as the depression rate increases. Mental health professionals advise parents to be aware of signs of depression in their children.

Some signs of depression in the teenager may be frequent sadness, crying or tearful spells, they may want to be alone most times and don't talk much. Teens may be writing poetry with morbid themes.

Self-Injury

Teens that have difficulty talking about their feelings may show their emotional tension, physical discomfort, pain and low self-esteem by cutting themselves.

They may feel hopeless like life is not worth living, do not take pride in their appearance and hygiene. They may also believe that a negative behavior will not change and so does not care about the future.

Children may drop out from activities they once enjoyed sometimes they even drop out of school.

They may live an isolated life and not willing to spend time with friends and families. Most of these children do not share their feelings as they feel no one is really listening to them and would not understand them.

There may be low energy and boredom in classes and so they miss classes and fail in school. These children often cause trouble at home or at school and not know they are depressed.

Parents do not think about their children being depressed and so a diagnosis of depression goes unnoticed. Parents are so busy trying to put a roof over their family and feed them that they hardly notice what is going on with their child.

These children are often depressed, angry or hostile with most of their anger projected towards their parents.

Sometimes teens may run away from home not because they want to run away but because they want help and do not know how to ask for it.

Because the child may not always seem sad, parents and teachers may not realize that the behavior problem is a sign of depression.

The teenager may talk about suicide or say things like they should be dead, or I want to kill myself, if you hear a child saying these things always take it seriously and seek help.

Some children may turn to drugs, alcohol and promiscuity, as a way out.

Treating the Depressed ADHD Teen

Early diagnosis is very important for the child. This may include medications counseling for both parents and child and other therapies. It is important that you follow through with the treatment. This could make a world of difference whether the child gets better or not.

Educating the Teen

When your child was first diagnosed with ADD/ADHD I am sure you received a lot of information concerning how to help your child. Now that your child has reached his/her teen years they need to understand the diagnosis and treatment and take responsibility for it. Therefore you need to educate your child about ADD/ADHD or have a caretaker educate them.

You should also educate the child about the outcome of negative attitudes and treatment.

Our children need knowledge and self confidence that he/she can take care themselves and this can only be gained by practice.

Time management

At this time your child should start learning about how to manage their time so they can take this into their teenage years and into adulthood. Help your child understand how to set an alarm clock so he/she can wake up on his/her own in the morning or have them wear a watch to check on the time they have to be back from a certain place. Give them the opportunity to be responsible.

Money Management

- Soon your teen will need to learn how to think of money as a means of gratification like buying that Mac Donald's or Chinese take out to learning how to budget for clothing, cell phone bill etc.

- One way to help your child learn how to manage money is by giving them a set allowance weekly, biweekly or monthly and have them put aside some of their savings to purchase something that they want. When children have to spend their own money they tend to look for bargains and spend wisely.

- They need to be educated on using a credit card wisely and saving for long term goals.

Organization

All children need to learn how to organize their belongings but the child that is diagnosed with ADD/ADHD has even more problems with this skill. Most teen keep their bedrooms, clothing and other things in a big mess that they can hardly find what they are looking for. I know some parents just close their child's bedroom door to avoid looking at a messy room.

Driving

Now that your teen has his/her driving license they will want to borrow your vehicle at times. They should be taught safety and what they should do in case of an emergency, like what to do if your car shuts down and it is dark, or if the car breaks down and you are far away from home.

Let them know that they need to call if they should be home at a certain time and they are not. Parents get very worried and they think the worst has happened.

Work with your child so they can gain confidence and responsibility.

- Teaching your teen to develop a filing system - Parents can help prepare their teen for this essential life management skill by developing a simple filing system for them during high school. At the beginning, it may be safer to file copies of essential information in your teen's personal file, keeping the originals safe in another location.

Personal Care

Now your child has to think about personal care which is a problem with teenagers .When your child was younger you reminded them to take care of or help them take care of their personal hygiene. These children have to be reminded at times to take care of their personal hygiene. Young children who do not learn to take care of themselves before leaving their parents house have a difficult time with the transition.

Sleep and the Teenager

The child that has ADD/ADHD has a difficult time sleeping especially when taking certain medications. Having a good night sleep is very important to function both at school and at home. They may need a cup of relaxing tea or a warm bath with some essential oil to help them unwind and fall asleep or some relaxing music.

Exercise and Nutrition

Exercise is very important and so is eating healthy. Help your child to understand what a healthy diet is about and encourage exercising. This helps reduce the impact of ADD/ADHD.

Social Skills

Children with ADD/ADHD have difficulty with social skills. Children practice social skills by copying what other grown up people do. These children with ADD/ADHD may miss learning these skills and have difficulty with being rejected and make fun of. Help is needed so that these children will be able to develop social skills.

Most teens may still be taking medications at this time and they need to know that they should find a way to remember to take their medication. Many teenagers believe that they do not need their medications at this time and they do not take it.

Some parents may decide to give their child behavioral intervention instead of medicines or any of the other treatments mentioned for children.

A child can live a successful life if their strengths are recognized and they are given the chance to prove themselves. There are many successful people with ADD/ADHD who never finished high school or college and went on to becoming successful people.

Even though your child is now a teen you need to let him/her know that he/she can still come to you with any problems and that you will be there to help them. Continue to let your child know that you still love them.

Alternative Treatment for ADHD

Attention Deficit Hyperactivity Disorder as stated before is often misdiagnosed which is frustrating for the child, the rest of the family, teachers and other healthcare professionals. Therefore everyone needs to work together in the best interest for the child.

I know how difficult it is to raise a child with ADHD and other health problems that go along with it. Believe me I have been in your shoes. There are lots of natural herbs you can use but you should seek the advice of a professional homeopathic or naturopathic doctor.

There are several natural treatment options which can be used alone or using more than one approach.

- Behavioral Approaches
- Cranio-Sacral therapy
- Karate
- Music
- Exercise
- Deep breathing

- Diet

- Meditation

- Yoga

- Faith

- Essential oils

- Energy healing

- Omega 3 Fatty Acids

- Magnesium with Vitamin D and Calcium

- Laughing

- Vitamin C it is vital in proper maintenance of the brain

- Multivitamins help improve the health of children. They help to prevent anemia and other diseases. You can find them in liquid form, chewable gummie bears or tablet form.

- Nature therapy

- Swimming

Behavior

Behavioral approach uses specific interventions that are goal oriented to change a particular behavior. They are used to provide structure and reinforce appropriate behaviors in the child with ADHD. Behavior interventions are used by parents, counselors, psychologists, school personnel and others.

Some behavioral approaches may include a token system where a child is given a token for a good behavior and have a token removed for inappropriate behavior. At the end of the day or at the end of the week decide if the child should earn something like an extra 30 minutes of TV, or 30 minutes of playing outside or a special treat. You can come up with your own treats.

You can also set time-outs for inappropriate behavior. You need to reinforce and let the child know when he/she did something appropriate also let them know when they did something inappropriate.

Cranio-sacral therapy

Try cranio-sacral therapy. This therapy involves the therapist placing their hands on the patient head. The practitioner gently works with the spine and the skull and its cranial sutures, diaphragms, and fascia. It is said this therapy eases the restrictions of nerve passages and the misaligned bones to be restored to their proper position. Cranio-sacral therapists use the therapy to treat mental stress, and other health problems.

Karate

Martial arts can be used to help the child focus and relieve impulsive behavior. It helps the c to improve the child mentally, physically and spiritually. It also helps to maintain health and develop their minds.

Music

Everyone loves music; music affects different parts of the brain. Most people love to listen to music especially when it is music that they love. Mozart, Beethoven and New Age music all help in retaining information, help with learning and communication skills.

Some children state that they study better when they have their favorite music playing. Mozart music also helps you to feel relaxed and calms hyperactivity.

When it is time for your child to get started on homework or for you to pay the bills maybe you should turn on the music.

Exercise

ADHD children need to have physical activities because they are full of energy. Games such as basketball, volleyball, running, swimming and other outdoor activities are great in helping the child burn off excess energy. These children should avoid sitting in front of the television and playing electronic games as a past time. Exercise is natural and inexpensive and can greatly help the ADHD child.

Deep breathing

Deep breathing help the child take in more oxygen into their body. A few deeps breaths does wonders for the body. If the child starts to feel dizzy for any reason stop the deep breathing and let the child sit and breathe normally. Deep breathing help relieve stress from the body.

Diet

Eating a high protein diet especially at breakfast help to improve concentration time. High protein foods include meat, beans, nuts and seed such as sunflower seeds, walnuts and almond nut.

- Eat complex carbohydrates like vegetables and fruits like pears, apples and kiwi.

- Eat less simple carbohydrates like products made from white sugar and white flour, candy, sodas and other foods with corn syrup.

- Eating more foods that contain Omega-3 fatty acids such as salmon, tuna and other cold water fish are said to be good for all but you need to take into consideration the mercury levels in the fish. Eating the younger fish seems to have less mercury. Walnuts and Brazil nuts are good sources of Omega-3 fatty acids.

Meditation

Children and adults who practice meditation twice a day for a t least 10 minutes find that they can focus better and are less stressed. Some schools in the United States are using meditation to help children focus better and in turn get better grades in school.

Younger children may not be able to meditate but they can try sitting quietly and undisturbed for a few minutes.

There are different types of meditation, sitting meditation, working meditation, walking meditation etc. If your child is old enough you can have them sit quietly in an erect position with the back not touching the wall or the back of the chair. Have the child breath in through the nose and count the breaths. Breathing in and out counts as one breath. They can count till 10 and the start from 1 again or they can pick a word that is suitable such as love, peace, Om or whatever word they may feel comfortable with sit quietly and repeat the same word for about 10-20 minutes depending on the age of the child.

Yoga (Super Brain Yoga)

According to reports in CBS2 News Super Brain Yoga has been shown to improve behavior performances and social skills in children with disabilities like ADD/ADHD.

Super Brain Yoga is a technique used to recharge and energize the brain. It uses the acupuncture sites of the lower ear lobes but does not use any needles. You use your hands instead and even small children can learn to do this. You can find for information on this by going to (CBS 2 News.com super brain power) or www.superbrainpower.com.

Faith

Everyone may not believe in faith and that is okay but I found faith helped me through the times when I struggled so much with my grandchild. Having a pastor or someone you can talk to who understands what you are going through makes a big difference. Just being able to talk to someone helps.

Essential Oils

Lavender

Lavender oil is good for almost everything. It also has a sedative and calming effect on both body and mind. Rub a few drops on the child's chest, temples, and feet can help relax them and help them to sleep more easily.

Cedar wood oil

This oil stimulates the function of the brain. Can be applied on the neck and forehead.

Frankincense

Help to improve mental function.

There are other oils that may be helpful.

A word of caution

Talk with your healthcare practitioner before use. Most oils need to be mixed with other base oils before use.

Energy healing

Reiki

Pronounced (rey-key) is the universal life energy. In some cultures it is known as chi, prana or spirit. Reiki channels the universal life energy to promote mental, spiritual and physical well-being. When used it is charging your batteries when they are low.

There are several different types of energy healing. You can Google energy healing www.energyhealing.com

Omega-3 fatty acids

Omega-3 fatty acid appears to be lower in most children diagnosed with ADD/ADHD. Parents may use flax seeds and or sea foods that have omega3 fatty acids. You can also supplement with Omega3 fish oils.

Magnesium Vitamin D and Calcium

Nutritional deficiencies are found in many children diagnosed with ADD/ADHD one of which is magnesium. Magnesium deficiency can be linked to calcium deficiency. Magnesium is thought to induce relaxation and help with thinking clearly and focusing.

Foods that include magnesium include:

Whole grain unrefined foods, seeds and nuts, black beans and tofu.

You may want to have you child tested for nutritional deficiencies before giving the magnesium, vitamin D and calcium or any other vitamins and minerals.

Stress

Find an outlet that can help you de-stress. Learning stress reduction techniques will help. Going for a walk out in nature can help you to calm down; gardening is another good tool, using stress balls which are round and about the size of golf balls. Stress balls are very cheap and effective.

Stress balls offer a psychological therapeutic value and this is achieved by causing distractions. When you hold a ball in each hand and start squeezing it, this takes your mind away from the stressor and in turn offers relief. This also tones the muscles of your hands and increases circulation in your blood stream. While travelling or standing in a long line, playing with these balls can also help pass time or at times calm you down when you are angry.

Small hard balls which are also called Chinese stress balls are rolled around the acupressure points in the palms of the hands. In addition to relieving stress they also clear the channels and strengthen the hands. They can be found in malls and in some Chinese stores.

Laughter

Laughter is the best medicine and it does not cost anything. It triggers healthy physical changes in the body, strengths the immune system and protect you from the damaging effects of stress. Laughter is fun, free and easy to use.

If you find it difficult to laugh especially after a stressful day, when you are in the shower no one is there listening to you so go ahead and even fake your laugh. It will do you a world of good.

Laughter has the power to heal and so does the mind.

Nature therapy

Nature therapy has been gaining momentum. In the book **"Last Child in the Woods: Saving Our Children from Nature-Deficit Disorder"** authored by Richard Louv talked about nature and the ADHD child. If where you live you cannot be in touch with nature a picture put up on the walls in the child's room may help tremendously or you can paint their room in green, or have green drapes in their room or a green sheet. Green is a calming color. *Studies have shown that children tend to be calmer and sleep better as a result of nature therapy or using green.*

Swimming

Since swimming needs a lot of focus and concentration these children do very well especially if they are to have individual attention.

Transformation Program: This is a program that help with behavior modification for defiant and out of control behavior by James Lehman.
I have not used this program personally but you may want to check it out.
The web is: www.totaltransformation.com/attention-deficit-disorder.aspx

So if you have a child, student, friend or anyone else who has been diagnosed with ADD/ADHD and having behavioral problems you may want to try this program.

Natural Treatment for ADHD

Attention Deficit Hyperactivity Disorder or ADHD affects 3-5% of all children. It is often misdiagnosed and treatment plans are not always effective.

The condition is frustrating for the child, the parent and the rest of the family. Teachers, physicians and other healthcare professionals become frustrated, as well. To achieve the best results, everyone in the child's environment needs to work together.

My goal here is to help you understand the condition and treatment options.

The most common symptoms of ADHD are impulsiveness, hyperactivity and inattention. Your child may not have all of these behavioral problems. Some kids are just hyperactive. Others get sidetracked, daydream or become bored, when they should be learning new skills.

Here are some casein-free foods rich in calcium and other minerals. If your child is deficient in calcium you may provide more of the foods listed below.

Vegetable sources:
Broccoli
Spinach
Turnip greens
Cabbage
Collard greens
Watercress
Bok choy
Brussels sprouts
Seaweed
Okra

Nuts and Legumes:
Peas
Peanuts
Almonds
Soy beans
Navy beans
Unhulled sesame seeds
White beans

Fish and seafood:
Sardines
Pink salmon
Mackerel
Shrimp

Other foods

Tofu
Corn
Corn tortillas
Blackstrap molasses

Although healthy and rich in vitamins and minerals, these casein-free foods may not be enough to meet your child's daily allowance of calcium. So you may want to give a calcium supplement to your child.

Supplemental Security Income (SSI)

Supplemental Security Income (SSI) is a federal program that provides assistance to people who have limited income and resources and who are at least 65 years old, or blind, or disabled under Social Security rules.

SSI is not just for adults. Children under the age of 18 years, who have disabilities, including some children with AD/HD, can receive SSI if they meet eligibility criteria.

The SSI program can provide monthly cash payments based on family income, the child can qualify for Medicaid health care services in many states, and ensure referral of a child into the system of care available under State Title V programs for Children with Special Health Care Needs.

Homeopathic Treatment versus Traditional Treatment

Homeopathic treatment helps ADHD children without resorting to potentially harmful drugs; the only drawback is that it takes longer to start seeing the effects. What steps should you take before deciding to use homeopathic treatment for an ADHD child?

- Confirm the ADHD diagnosis with appropriate evaluations.

- Research all available treatment options – both conventional medicine and homeopathy.

- Evaluate the benefits and risks of treatments and select the treatment best suited to your child.

- Choose credible reputable professionals with demonstrated success in treating ADHD children.

- Form a team consisting of your family, health care professionals, and homeopathic practitioner.

- Write a contract committing the group to work together for specified goals for helping the ADHD child.

76

- Evaluate treatment results regularly – every six months is a good milestone.

- Modify treatment plans as necessary to achieve the desired results for your ADHD child.

By combining homeopathic remedies, modification of diet and behavior management may yield best results for your child without the side effects of long term medications. Until your child is ready to accept and change his/her ways and thinking no amount of counseling will help.

Dr. Amen is an Assistant Clinical Professor of Psychiatry and Human Behavior at the University of California, Irvine School of Medicine, where he teaches medical students and psychiatric residents about using brain imaging in clinical practice.

Daniel G. Amen, MD is a physician, child and adult psychiatrist, brain imaging specialist, bestselling author, Distinguished Fellow of the American Psychiatric Association and the CEO and medical director of Amen Clinics, Inc. (ACI) in Newport Beach and Fairfield, California, USA. Tacoma, Washington, USA and Reston, Virginia, USA .

Dr. Amen has written several books including Change Your Brain, Change Your Life, Magnificent Mind at Any Age, Healing ADD, Making A Good Brain Great and many others. Dr Amen uses special scans to determine what part of the brain is not functioning as it should and how to treat it. He uses mostly natural supplements to treat the specific part of the brain.

His clinics are based in California, Virginia and New York, USA.

Phone 1 949 266 3700
www.amenclinics.com

Anger and ADHD

Many children diagnosed with ADD/ADHD may have feelings of anger which can be very difficult for them to manage. Stressful and frustrating situations usually cause intense anger. These children have a hard time stopping to think about how to react to certain situations so they quickly lose control of themselves.

Look for triggers in your child example when they are too tired, certain times of the day like when they get home from school, when they eat certain foods, when hungry or if the medication is wearing off.

When you see your child getting angry try to intervene very calmly before it becomes full blown. Depending on the age of your child you can probably give a back rub, a hug or take a few deep breaths together with your child and count to 10. This may help calm them down.

Help your child to understand the situation and how to analyze it before reacting. You can role play with your child to help them understand the situation.
These children when they want something they want it now and does not know how think that if I can't get it now maybe I can get it later.

You may need to have your child be seen by a counselor to help him/her deal with anger, to evaluate their feelings and how to react to a situation.

CHADD

The <u>National Resource Center on ADHD: A Program of CHADD</u> is the nation's clearinghouse for science-based information about all aspects of attention-deficit/hyperactivity disorder (ADHD). Funded by the Centers for Disease Control and Prevention, the NRC provides information on this disorder which affects how millions of children and adults function on a daily basis.

You can join CHADD by going to www. CHADD.org. You can also get useful information such as locating a chapter near you.

Taking Care of Yourself

It is very important that you take care of yourself. Because these children wear you out you have to be strong to be there to help them. Sometimes parents think they are so tired with dealing with the child and other siblings plus taking care of the household and also a job they do not have the time or energy to care of themselves. If you continue this way you would need your child or someone else to take care of you instead.

Some things you can do for yourself that is very cost effective are:

Have an older sibling that is capable of caring for the younger ones for an evening where you and your partner can go out to eat or go to the movies and enjoy an evening together alone.

Take sometime of and prepare a nice hot bath with some essential oils, light a candle and play some soft music without being disturbed.

Or if you have a friend with children you can take turns watching the children one evening for the week or hire a baby sitter for an evening.

I am sure you can come up with some other very inexpensive ways to spend an evening away from your child/children to restore yourself.

Always make sure if you are leaving your child/children with someone, that they can easily contact you in case of an emergency.

In some areas there is an organization called "RESPITE" if there is one in your area you may want to take advantage of it. It is a place where you can leave your child for a few hours so that you can take a break.

My personal experience. For several years I was overstressed with caring for my ADHD grandchild and was also working full time. Then I moved to another state and stress took over my life. I could not concentrate any more on what I was doing and so had to give up my job.

I did not know anything about relieving stress and so I suffered in silence. Then about one year after I moved a Buddhist temple opened in my neighborhood and out of curiosity I visited it, everyone in the temple was very nice and invited myself and my family to their service.

We did go to the service, my family and I still attend their services after several years. That was three years ago. What I have learned there turned my life around. I am not saying that I do not get stressed but I learned how to control it and let it go. Stress does not control me anymore. I feel so much better.

Putting it together. I hope that you will find the information that is given in eBook very helpful. I have personally used many of them which helped in some ways.

My advice to you before using any of the information in this book that you have your child evaluated and diagnosed by a professional clinician and let them know what you will be using for your child if you choose not to medicate your child.

Using any of the information in this eBook without proper advice from your medical doctor is at your own risk. The information in this eBook is for informational purposes only. Your child may feel better but not cured.

Resources

www.nlcd.com

www.chadd.org

www.superbrainyoga.com

www.energyhealing.com

www.adhd.com

www.adhdandteens.com

www.naturaltreatmentforadhd.com

www.meditation.com

www.amensclinic.com

www.totaltransformation.com

www.ingramcontent.com/pod-product-compliance
Lightning Source LLC
Chambersburg PA
CBHW070551290526
45790CB00002B/647